DIABETES

DIABETES: REVERSE TYPE 2 DIABETES, LOWER YOUR BLOOD SUGAR, AND LIVE A HEALTHIER LIFE IN 12 SIMPLE STEPS

Disclaimer

This book is only intended as an informational guideline to help reverse type-2 diabetes, and should not be considered expert instruction. All attempts have been made to verify the information listed in this book; however, the author cannot assume any responsibility for any loss, damage or misappropriation of any information herein contained.

Always consult your healthcare practitioner before starting a new meal or exercise plan.

Introduction

Take control of your health!

Type-2 diabetes is *reversible.*

Take a moment. Let that sink in.

Now think about this: type-2 diabetes is caused by eating too many carbs, which leads to the body producing too much insulin and eventually becoming resistant to it. And how do we treat this disease? With *more* insulin! And while we're treating the *symptoms* of diabetes, the *underlying problem* of insulin resistance is left to progress. Type-2 diabetes is only a chronic progressive disease because it's not being treated correctly – we need to treat the underlying problem, not just its symptoms. And the underlying problem is eating too much of the wrong foods.

The answer then is simple: take control of this disease by taking control of your diet. With some diligence and consistency, you can get your body back into a metabolically healthy state in which it is more than capable of controlling its own insulin levels – before it's too late.

So, now that we've got these simple (yet life-changing) facts out of the way, let's get into the nitty-gritty about how to accomplish it. Because yes, it's within your power to take control of your body and health, and give yourself the gift of good quality of life. And in the end, throwing all that medication in the dustbin where it belongs.

So are you ready to tackle diabetes head-on? Let's get started!

Contents

Chapter 1
Treat the disease, not the symptoms

"You are what you eat."

This often-uttered statement is old news. But it's also one of the most significant, and truest, things you'll ever hear about your health. The sad thing is that because it's become such a wrung-out old saying, no one really gives it a second thought anymore.

But let's start at the beginning. In recent decades, after thousands of years of having a good handle on nutrition, we seem to have lost our way. Processed foods became staples in our diet. Instead of healthy, nutritious food, we now eat refined carbohydrates that have no nutritional value. The refined sugar industry is *booming* (160 million tons of sugar is produced annually).

In this same period of time, public health started a steady decline, as obesity and type-2 diabetes started an ascent as two of the most common health problems of this century – along with a slew of other diseases (heart disease, cancer). And our response has been to treat diabetes with insulin, and obesity with eating less and moving more. This may seem logical, but in effect, diabetes as well as obesity are only symptoms of a bigger problem. And if you want to fix a problem, you need to start treating it, rather than its symptoms.

So what is the problem? "We are what we eat."

Our bodies aren't equipped to deal with what we're putting into them – and we rarely even know what that is. We eat food that has been prepared by someone else – in the form of take-aways, restaurants, and about 90% of the grocery store. And these foods are all full of chemicals, preservatives, sugar and unhealthy fat parading as food. We have to realise that these processed foods are manufactured by companies who are focused on a bottom line – not consumer health. Adding a chemical that makes something taste like fruit is a lot more cost-effective than adding the actual fruit. And so, these products have become diluted with cheap alternatives, chemicals to make them taste better, preservatives to make them last for years, and astounding doses of sugar and salt to make them yummy – completely empty, nutrient-less calories. The result is food items with ingredient lists that read like lab reports. Even applying the word "food" to these products is stretching it.

So with this in mind, is it really any wonder we're getting sicker and fatter?

But nobody has to be a victim of type-2 diabetes. Not only is it preventable, but it is also reversible. All you need to do is take your health and your diet into your own hands.

Chapter 2
A step-by-step guide to reverse diabetes

Diabetes and pre-diabetes cost America $322 billion per year

These 12 simple steps are designed to get you going in the right direction – they have everything you need to get clued up and take on a practical approach towards reversing diabetes. All you need to do is read them!

Step 1: Get your mindset right

The World Health Organisation projects that diabetes will be the seventh leading cause of death in 2030

It's so important to realise the power of having the right mindset. One that will keep you motivated, even when it feels like you aren't making progress. This is the cornerstone to effecting real change in your life. Once determination has gotten a hold of you, it's so much easier to wake up every morning positive and knowing the day will be a success.

So change your mindset. Take on the challenge to change your health. It can be done, you just need to go ahead and do it. Once you've gotten yourself into the right headspace, there's nothing that will feel too daunting for you. And once you start seeing those changes in your health, it will only add fuel to your fire.

Step 2: Understand what's going on inside your body

"The number of people with diabetes has risen from 108 million in 1980 to 422 million in 2014"
– The World Health Organisation

Traditionally, medical science has been stuck on outdated knowledge of the workings of the human body. It might seem odd in this day and age, but how our bodies really work is extremely complex. So, the idea behind taking more insulin to regulate blood sugar has been predicated on beliefs that we cannot lower carb intake, as our bodies and brains are too dependent on glucose (from carbs) for energy. Within that, it was believed, and still widely is, that we need at least 120g of carbs every day just for the brain to function optimally. But what we now know is that the brain and body can function fantastically well on fat for energy, and the body can create its own glucose in a process called gluconeogenesis. In fact, many are saying that we don't need any carbs *at all*. But this doesn't mean that you should cut out all your carbs! Fruits and vegetables are where you get many of your vitamins and minerals from – a God-given health tonic straight from nature.

Unfortunately, it seems that many sufferers of diabetes do not know the simple science behind it, or are still hanging on to outdated information. But we're about to change that. To better understand type-2 diabetes, you have to understand your body's response to food. Insulin is the most important part of this.

The insulin effect

When you take in carbohydrates, the body breaks them down into glucose (sugar). Many people still think you only find sugar in candy, so reduce the sweet stuff and you're sorted. But this simply isn't true. It is not only people with a sweet tooth who develop this disease. It doesn't matter what kind of carb you eat: pasta, bread, "healthy" cereal – they all get broken down into sugar.

Carbs are quickly metabolised, unlike fat and most proteins. The result is glucose (which your body can now use for energy) flooding the bloodstream: high blood sugar. Since this is bad for the body and gunks up the system, the body releases insulin in response. This hormone binds to the insulin receptors on your muscle, liver and fat cells, which then allows the cells to take in the glucose. Additionally, insulin prompts the body to store glucose as fat, which is why type-2 diabetes is usually associated with being overweight. Clearly, this is a very important hormone.

Insulin resistance

Over time, the body can start to develop resistance to something. Think about alcohol or sugar. The first drink you ever had might've gotten you drunk, but now your tolerance for alcohol is much higher. If you don't take sugar in your tea or coffee, it will taste a bit sickly to you if someone serves you a sugary cup. However, if you gradually added more sugar, you would eventually get used to it, and coffee would taste bitter to you without the added sweetness.

This principle is exactly the same for your body and insulin. Your cells start developing a resistance to insulin, and your body has to secrete more and more to get those cells to open up and take in the glucose.

This can cause a bit of a snowball effect when you often eat food that is high in processed carbohydrates, because they have been stripped of the fibre found in natural whole foods which slows down digestion and consequently the flooding of glucose into the bloodstream. The body continually has to up its insulin production, and you start getting insulin resistant.

But why don't the cells want more energy? Because they're getting way more than they need. While processed foods are nutrient poor, they are energy (calorie) dense. The result is that we keep plying our bodies with energy that we simply don't use. Glucose is the type of energy your body might want for strenuous physical activity, because it's more readily available than your fat stores (fat has to be metabolised for energy). But if you're sitting at a desk all day, barely doing anything more physically demanding than walking to the kitchen to get a cup of coffee, you really don't need all this quick-absorbing sugar, as your body has nothing to do with it. Eating massive amounts of carbs is like hooking yourself up to an energy IV. The result is cells that are, quite frankly, sick of taking up so much energy.

Insulin resistance is the first step towards pre-diabetes. At this point, the process leading to full-blown type-2 diabetes has been kick-started.

Pre-diabetes

With pre-diabetes, the blood sugar levels are elevated, but not yet at the point where it qualifies as full-blown diabetes.

Type-2 diabetes

When your body has been put through the wringer like this, it eventually reaches a point where it can no longer properly control its own insulin levels, and it needs medical help to do so. This is called type-2 diabetes. As the body struggles to regulate its insulin, numerous complications start appearing, from blurred vision, fatigue and headaches to limb amputations, blindness and death. It is a very serious disease.

Type-1 vs type-2

It might be interesting to note at this point where type-1 diabetes fits into the picture. This kind of diabetes is also known as juvenile diabetes, as it usually rears its head in childhood and early adulthood. However, it also occurs in adults. Only 5% of people with diabetes have type-1.

Type-1 diabetes occurs when your immune system attacks and destroys your insulin-making beta cells, which are located in the pancreas. This then impairs the body's ability to produce insulin, so that there is not enough to allow the cells to take up glucose, leaving them without energy. This leads to high blood sugar, as all that glucose is now floating around in the bloodstream. In addition, it also impairs the body's ability to stop producing its own sugar (gluconeogenesis). So while type-2 is a result of too much insulin, type-1 is a result of too little insulin.

Step 3: Become a nutrition know-it-all

The three macro-nutrients

For our bodies to function properly, we need three basic macro-nutrients (commonly referred to as macros): carbs, protein and fat. Each of these fulfils important roles within our bodies. It has been the tendency to vilify some of these macros in attempts to find the perfect diet – just like low fat used to be all the rage, the tide is now turning towards low carb. In truth, it's much more about finding balance within these macros and not forgetting those all-important micro-nutrients – vitamins and minerals.

Carbohydrates

Insulin effect: High

Complex (healthy) carbs: *Green and starchy vegetables, legumes, lentils, brown rice, oatmeal, beans*

Simple (unhealthy) carbs: *Refined sugar, candy, soft drinks, milk and milk products, fruit juice (fibre is removed in the juicing process), syrup, high-fructose corn syrup (added to many processed foods), white bread, baked goods, pasta*

There are two types of carbohydrates: simple and complex. Simple carbs consist of shorter chains of molecules that are easier for your body to break down and consequently are absorbed into the bloodstream much quicker. Complex carbs consist of longer chains and are more difficult for your body to break down, and are consequently absorbed slower, causing less of a blood sugar spike.

Carbohydrates are made up of three components: sugar, starch and fibre. Fibre and starch are complex carbs, and sugar is a simple carb.

While whole fruits can be classified as simple carbs, they have lots of fibre as well, slowing down the digestion process.

All carbs are eventually broken down and converted by the body into glucose (sugar). Glucose travels to the liver and is distributed to the cells in the tissue and muscle. Your body stores some glucose in the muscles and liver as glycogen, but the amount it is capable of storing here is finite (about 400g, depending on your size), and the rest that your body doesn't use is stored as fat.

Your body uses glucose for energy, and it is the most efficient source of energy for the body, since it is readily available and easily used by the cells. This is why when it comes to peak performance and high-intensity exercise, glucose helps you to perform your best. Traditionally, this has been why athletes carb-load and are so dependent on carbs for performance. However, recent research has indicated the benefits of fat as the best source of sustainable energy.

The problem with a high-carb diet for the average person who spends most of their time sedentary, seated in front of a computer, is then quite obvious – they do not use almost any of this influx of carbs, resulting in most of it just being stored in the body as fat.

It is in this super-fast absorbency that we see the biggest problem with consuming high-calorie, nutrient-poor simple carbs (like bread). They are just not satisfying for the body, because all they do is spike insulin without providing any nutritional benefits. Studies have even shown that consuming something sugary before a meal, like a soft drink, can actually make you eat more.

Because insulin needs to be released for the cells to take up all this glucose, the body is not able to use stored body fat as energy. As mentioned before, insulin is a fat-storage hormone, so that any excess glucose that the body doesn't want just floating around can be converted into fat and safely stored. The body is thus in fat-storage mode, as opposed to fat-burning mode.

As the blood sugar drops rapidly because the insulin is getting rid of the glucose and the body can't easily access stored fat, the brain starts signalling for more carbs in the form of cravings – specifically bad carbs with high sugar loads, because sugar also triggers a dopamine response. Have you ever noticed how you crave pizza or chocolate, but not broccoli or steamed fish fillets? It's the body's dependency on carbs that's rearing its ugly head, and this is the only reason why people overeat. People are not overweight because they can't control themselves around food. They're overweight because they're eating the wrong kinds of foods, leading to an unhealthy metabolic system, of which obesity and diabetes are just some of the symptoms.

Why your body needs carbs

Unlike the essential amino acids and essential fatty acids we get from protein and fat respectively, because our bodies can't make their own, there is nothing essential that we get from carbs, because we can make our own glucose (gluconeogenesis). This is why many health practitioners have started advocating the idea the carbs are completely unnecessary. However, natural carbs like fruits and vegetables are packed with micro-nutrients, which keep you healthy and functioning optimally. It is very unfortunate that so many people are losing sight of this.

Fat

Insulin effect: Low

Healthy fats: *Avocados, nuts and seeds, coconut oil, olive oil, olives, grass-fed butter, oily fish like salmon, natural nut butters, high-cacao dark chocolate (80% and higher)*

Unhealthy fats: *Trans fats found in fast foods, deep-fried foods, margarine, hydrogenated vegetable oils*

We already know that the body also uses stored fat as a source of energy, and recent research has seen high-fat diets gain popularity. Because fat is so much harder to break down, it provides a much more stable energy source. It is also much more filling, and helps to fight cravings for unhealthy carb-based foods. This is why the ketogenic diet was formulated, which consists of mostly fat: about 80% fat, 15% protein, 5% carb. The idea with this diet is to keep your carb intake low enough that your insulin remains low and your body can naturally go into ketosis (running on stored fat for energy). When your body is already insulin resistant, it can take a while for the body to naturally adjust to this.

While it is true that fat is filling, it is also much more energy-dense than carbs and protein. Fat is about 9 calories per gram, while carbs and protein are 4 calories per gram.

Why your body needs fat

Fat contains essential fatty acids that cannot be made by the body for growth and cell function. It also supports brain function and prompts the release of leptin – the satiety hormone (vs ghrelin, the hunger hormone). Leptin makes you feel full and signals the body to stop eating. In addition, some vitamins are fat-soluble: vitamins A, D, E and K.

Protein

Insulin effect: Moderate

Healthy proteins: *Fish, chicken, red meats, quinoa, eggs*

Unhealthy proteins: *Processed meats like sausages, sandwich meats, fast foods*

While carbs have a huge impact on insulin levels, and fat makes almost no noticeable difference, protein falls somewhere in the middle. Accordingly, it should not be consumed without accompanying fibrous vegetables and fat.

Why your body needs protein

Protein is incredibly important for the body, specifically its essential amino acids (which cannot be made by the body). While protein occurs naturally in fruits and vegetables as well, these often don't feature the complete chain of amino acids in sufficient amounts, like meat and eggs do. So for vegetarians and vegans, it's important to eat a varied diet to get enough of the essential amino acids. Pairing different foods like rice (grains) with beans (legumes) gives the complete chain of amino acids in sufficient amounts.

How do I know how much of which macro I'm eating?

If you want to know how much of which macro you're consuming, you'll need to look up a particular food's nutritional info, and then weigh the food to determine how much of what it has. For example, if you google the nutritional value of a chicken fillet, you'll find that it contains per 100g:

14g of fat, 0g of carbs and 27g of protein. So, if you're eating a chicken fillet that weighs 150g, the macro breakdown will be as follows: 21g fat, 0g carbs and 40.5 protein.

Needless to say, this can be quite tedious to do every day, but luckily there are many apps on the market that can help you track your macros and that have food databases so you don't have to look everything up. It's immensely helpful to work out a weekly mealplan and prepare accordingly beforehand, so you don't have to weigh everything you eat during the week.

Step 4: Eat to reverse diabetes

TIP: Apple cider vinegar has been shown to have blood sugar stabilising effects and blunt cravings for sugar

---

Now that you have a better handle on how insulin operates in the body and how the three basic macro-nutrients affect the process, it's time to start implementing that into your eating.

And so we get to the dreaded part: diet. This word is hated by so many people, but it's time to start thinking about it differently. The human body is a wonderfully complicated system; something that allows us to physically function within our world. So much of our quality of life is dependent upon the efficient running of this system. Our bodies are our most valuable possessions – something that could never be replaced. And we need to treat them as such. That's why what we put into our bodies is so important, because you do get out what you put in.

However, I want to throw the word "diet" out of the equation, and replace it with the concept of a "way of eating". Because that's all it is. When you feed your body the right stuff, your metabolic health and your weight will all fall into place. The human body is perfectly capable of regulating its own weight and keeping itself healthy and functioning optimally. We just need to give it the right tools. This helps us to build healthier relationships with food. It shouldn't be something to fear or avoid, or something that has power over you.

Here are some rules to live by in order to start reversing your body's diabetes:

Manage your weight

Obesity and type-2 diabetes tend to be linked, but it's not entirely clear why having excess fat cells makes you more prone to developing type-2 diabetes. What we do know is that fat cells produce hormones that interfere with insulin, leading to insulin resistance. But it is clear that reducing your weight is very effective for reversing insulin resistance.

In order to manage your body weight, it's worth figuring out how many calories you need to be consuming every day. There are many calculators online that can work this out for you. It consists of two things: your basal metabolic rate (BMR) and your activity level (how active your job is and how much you exercise). Your BMR is how many calories your body needs in a day even when you're just sitting in front of the computer. Your body needs calories for all its internal processes (like breathing). Otherwise, an activity tracker can give you an estimate of how many calories you burn during a day. These are all just estimates, however, and it's impossible to really know what your BMR is or how many calories you burn when you're active.

If you would like to lose some weight, a healthy caloric deficit to be in is about 200 to 500 calories. Anything more than that and the body will start thinking it's starving and hold on tightly to fat. Often people who drastically restrict calories when dieting lose a lot of weight, but half of it is muscle. All this does is slow down the metabolism, so when you start eating normally again, you will regain the weight quite quickly, and sometimes even some more.

If you eat healthy for long enough, your body will eventually fall into a comfortable weight that's natural and healthy for you. Counting calories is not meant to be a permanent thing. Once you have done it for a while, you will learn what an appropriate portion size is, and naturally eat correctly.

Eat real food

If you're not naturally good cook, it might be worth investing in some cookbooks to get you going.

Real food – whole, one-ingredient foods from the earth – is what your body wants to eat; what it was made to eat. By far the majority of the foods in supermarkets today are very, very processed. Any time food is processed to make something new, it is essentially being tampered with, and in almost all cases, losing any health benefits.

Let's take an example: wheat. This is *the* staple of the Western diet. It's in bread, pasta, cereal, baked goods. Originally, maybe a hundred years ago, before wheat was bred to be a staple food for entire populations, it looked much different to how it does now, and it was much more nutritious. But since then, it has been bred to grow faster and be bigger, since this industry is profit-driven, like any other. The more plant you get per yield, the better. And if it can be done cheaper, even better. Today, wheat no longer looks like it did a hundred years ago, and has lost much of its nutritional value.

Then comes the refining process. The wheat is stripped, and the plant loses about 90% of its nutrients, and its fibre. It's now a raw product ready to be made into bread, for instance. During this process, the wheat flour is added to in order to make bread – but what are they adding? Mostly chemicals and preservatives. In addition, they might try to fortify it with some vitamins. It's highly unlikely that those vitamins will be absorbed by your body. So the end product, a slice of bread, offers you no nutritional benefits whatsoever.

In this case, you might opt for whole-wheat. Because, if they use the whole-grain, instead of cutting away the nutritious bit, it must be okay to eat, right? Unfortunately, it's not that easy. It might say "whole-grain" on the packet, but it's actually only partially so.

This does not mean to say that everything that comes out of a packet is bad. There are definitely healthy alternatives. For instance, regular peanut butter versus natural peanut butter – if you look on the label and it reads like a lab experiment, you know it's unhealthy, but if the only ingredient listed is peanuts, you're good to go. Learn to read labels, and at the very least just pick the healthy version of something.

Where possible, always eat organic. It's free of pesticides and hormones that can mess with your own hormones.

Focus on your macro intake

You have to get your refined-carb intake under control, in order to get out of the vicious cycle of hunger, cravings and fat storage, and the resultant blood sugar ups and downs.

This means eating low carb and high fat. Because of long-instilled prejudice against fat, this might cause you a fair amount of panic. But as we've discussed in Step 3, fat is a good thing, and it certainly isn't going to expand your waistline – that's sugar's job. But here comes a big BUT: don't just lose all self-control and eat any form of fat you can get a hold on. All those extra calories can up your weight.

If you've worked out your ideal caloric intake, you can work out what your macro split should be and how much of which macro you should be eating. If your total daily calories is 1600 and you want to stick to the low-carb, high-fat approach, you'll want something like the ketogenic macro split: 80% fat, 15% protein, 5% carb. This gives you the following number of calories you need to consume of each macro-nutrient:

Fat: 80% of 1600 = 1280 calories from fat

Protein: 15% of 1600 = 240 calories from protein

Carbs: 5% of 1600 = 80 calories from carbs

You can then work out how many grams of each you need:

Fat: 1280 calories ÷ 9 calories per gram of fat = 142g of fat

Protein: 240 calories ÷ 4 calories per gram of protein = 60g of protein

Carbs: 80 calories ÷ 4 calories per gram of carbs = 20g of carbs

The ketogenic approach is very low in carbs, and this might be excessive for some people. You can also eat up to 40 or even 60 grams of carbs and still consider it a low-carb diet. Even though this sounds like a very little, you could eat an entire salad made up of low-carb vegetables and be under your carb count. It needs to be emphasised that low-carb doesn't mean zero carb. While refined sugars and grains deliver truckloads of glucose into the bloodstream, fruits and vegetables don't have the same effect. Healthy foods are also much lower in calories.

Find what works best for you. As you become more insulin sensitive, you will be able to eat more carbs and not have it be such a detrimental effect on your health.

Here's a list with some examples of diabetes-friendly foods:

Low-carb wholefoods

Always eat organic and/or free range as far as possible – these foods are pesticide and hormone free

This list is by no means comprehensive, and the golden rule is always natural is better than processed. If you are unsure about the carb content of a fruit, google it. Try to stick to fruits that don't contain multiple teaspoons of sugar (4g = 1 tsp) per 100g

Leafy greens

Packed with nutrients and very low in calories, most leafy greens and some other veggies are considered "free foods" (you don't need to count their calories as part of your total)

Spinach	Kale
Swiss chard	Cabbage
Broccoli	Rocket
Lettuce	Brussels sprouts
Cauliflower	

Other veggies

Veggies are naturally low in sugars and pack a lot of nutrients for their weight

Zucchini	Carrots
Asparagus	Garlic
Artichokes	Red onion
Eggplant	Tomatoes
Paprika	Red pepper
Cucumber	Olives
Celery	Radish
Jalapeno peppers	

Eat balanced meals

The different macros in the foods we eat do affect one another once they have entered the body. If you simply eat a very lean cut of meat, with no fat or fibre to slow down digestion of the food, the resulting insulin load can be very heavy. Remember, meat also prompts insulin to some degree. Similarly, you want fat present at every meal to slow the digestion process.

This is why it's so important to make sure your meals are balanced.

Step 5: Do intermittent fasting

Human beings have been fasting for thousands of years! It's a very natural thing for our bodies.

What is intermittent fasting?

It consists of two parts: eating and not eating (ie fasting). This is already what you do every day when you go to sleep. All that happens with intermittent fasting is that the eating window is made shorter, while the fasting window is made longer.

Fasting has been around for thousands of years, in many different forms, and people still do it today. We commonly recognise it as a religious practice.

But in this context, fasting doesn't refer to going without food for days at a time. Instead, the focus is on fasting for a period throughout the day. How long this period is, is completely up to the individual and what works for them.

However, the 16/8 split is probably the most common: 16 hours of fasting and eight hours of eating. More aggressive approaches might be 18/6 or even 20/4. Some people go as far as to only eat one meal a day. You could also try fasting for a few days at a time to accelerate the process.

It takes the body about 12 hours to burn through its glucose and glycogen stores, at which point it will become reliant on fat for energy. At this point insulin levels are reduced to zero. Fasting is the most effective way to reduce insulin. While a low-carb diet, like the ketogenic diet, will reduce carb intake, it is fasting that will reduce insulin levels.

Debunking common myths about fasting

"Breakfast, lunch and dinner"

Intermittent fasting has been doing the rounds lately, especially among the fitness crowd, but for many people it is still an alien concept. The first response to fasting is that it must surely be unhealthy to skip meals. From a young age, we are taught that breakfast, lunch and dinner are firm fixtures, with breakfast being the most important meal of the day to jump-start the metabolism, and some snacks in between keeping the metabolism going. In truth, the three meals a day with snacks idea is a wholly manmade concept. There really is no reason that you have to eat at 7am, 1pm or 7pm. Your body is perfectly capable of going without food for periods of time. Have you ever woken up faint and light-headed because your body had to endure eight hours without food when sleeping? Not likely. Few people even get hungry in the early morning.

"Snack to keep the metabolism going"

It's the same with eating a snack in between meals to keep the metabolism going. The momentary increase in metabolism that burns more calories won't even make a dent in the number of calories contained in the snack. What's more, if you're eating the right types of food – balanced meals with healthy fat, protein and fibre – you shouldn't be hungry for many hours after you've eaten – up to five or six.

"Breakfast is the most important meal of the day"

Ideas like "breakfast is the most important meal of the day" are mostly perpetuated by food companies wanting to sell their products, and these products are usually ridiculously unhealthy. Take something like cereal, bagels or muffins – all traditionally acceptable breakfast foods. But they contain no nutritional value, and just dump large amounts of sugar into the bloodstream. Muffins are essentially cupcakes without any icing on them – they have the same ingredients. And the so-called "healthier" bran or blueberry muffins are even worse, because they have that much more sugar in them to make them taste better. The "blue things" they put in blueberries are in many cases not even real blueberries. So ask yourself again: does this sound like a healthy start to the day? Dumping numerous teaspoons of sugar into the bloodstream, with no nutritional benefit?

"Starvation mode"

Another myth is that you cannot go without calories for long periods of time, as your body will go into "starvation mode". But this only happens when you eat fewer total daily calories. With intermittent fasting, you are still eating the same total daily calories, just in a shorter window of time.

As mentioned before, every time we eat, our blood sugar spikes. This isn't just true of eating carbs: fat and protein also play their part. And for those with insulin resistance, pre-diabetes and type-2 diabetes, it happens uncontrollably.

The logical reasoning then would be to eat less frequently, giving the body more time to recover its equilibrium and get into the habit of burning fat for energy.

Benefits of fasting

Increased energy

Because the body is no longer subject to the energy ups and downs that come with sugar intake and the resultant insulin spikes, your energy levels are stable when fasting. They don't dip up and down, because the body is coasting along in ketosis (burning fat for energy). Adrenaline levels also go up in the fasted state, leading to increased energy.

Increased mental clarity

This is often cited as one of the best benefits of fasting. In a fasted state, it is often much easier to concentrate. The reason is quite simply because less time and resources have to be spent on digestion by the body, allowing sharper mental focus on the task at hand. Additionally, because you know you won't be eating, you are less likely to be thinking about what you could be snacking on.

Healing

When the body spends less time constantly digesting, it also has more time to focus on other pursuits, like cell repair. Therapeutic fasting (fasting for multiple days and consuming only water) isn't only used to treat diabetes, it is also used to treat high blood pressure, lupus, rheumatoid arthritis and psoriasis, among others.

Longevity

Studies have shown that eating less and less often can extend life and slow the ageing process.

Growth hormone

Fasting increases growth hormone in the body, which preserves lean muscle. In other words, you don't have to worry about losing muscle instead of fat when fasting for extended periods.

You can eat bigger meals

As mentioned before, you only go into starvation mode of you severely restrict your calories, so don't eat fewer calories when you fast. The goal is to eat the same amount as you usually would, your meals are just going to be bigger. Instead of having to worry about restricting your calories, the problem is then more often to get in enough. Besides the fat-burning benefits, this is also one of the benefits of intermittent fasting for weight loss.

Where to start

It's not necessary to dive head-long into fasting for a prolonged part of the day. There really are no set rules – you don't have to begin or stop eating on the hour. It doesn't have to be any particular time of day either. Let's say, for instance, your fasting window is 16 hours and your eating window is eight hours. The fasting window can begin right after your last meal or snack of the day, for example 9pm. Or you could eat during the morning and early afternoon, and fast during the evening. Note that if you follow an exercise programme (see Step 7), you'll want to consume a balanced meal afterwards to give your body the nutrients it needs to repair your muscles – especially protein and carbs.

Tips for fasting beginners

1. Begin with a shorter fasting window and work up to a longer one.
2. Drink lots of water – it'll fill you up.
3. Drink black coffee or tea – it has an appetite-suppressing effect but is still low enough in calories that it doesn't have much of an effect on insulin.

Step 6: Form good habits and ditch bad ones

Nutrition

To overhaul your entire diet won't be easy – at first. It is, after all, something you've spent many years doing a certain way. Convenience foods are convenient, and they make our busy lives much easier. But I want to tell you that eating for good health instead of eating what's easy and immediately satisfying is something that eventually becomes habit.

Set yourself up for success by starting early in the morning, with something like a big glass of water and some black coffee. If you're not fasting in the morning, eat a healthy breakfast. This will get you on track for the rest of the day, and make it easier to stick to your mealplan.

If you have a cheat meal every now and then, try to have it on a Sunday, as it's much easier to get back on the mealplan on a Monday, rather than still having the entire weekend ahead.

It's also a good idea to stock up on healthy foods, especially healthy snacks. This makes it so much easier to make better choices. Usually, the only way to get hold of healthy snacks is to make them. This can be something you do on one particular day every week.

If you spend a lot of time at the office, consider preparing food in advance as well, to make your week that much easier.

These are the types of things that may seem like a lot of effort at first, but in time, if you diligently do it, it will become habit to the point where you don't really have to think about it that much anymore. This will ultimately make life much easier for you.

Sleep

Getting a good eight hours of sleep is very important to maintain healthy hormone levels, and it's worth it to get a good routine down to aid in getting quality sleep. If your body is used to a certain before-bed routine, getting some good sleep becomes easier. Obviously this involves keeping to the same bedtime every night. Also get into the habit of winding down before bedtime, like reading a book instead of watching TV, as the blue light emitted from electronic screens mimic daylight and confuse the body's natural rhythms.

You can also do something relaxing like taking a hot shower or bath – or even a cold one. This has also been shown to promote better sleep.

Exercise

With exercise, it's also all about routine. For most people, it's easier to work out in the mornings, as that way they're more likely to do it. This depends on the individual though, but try to get a set time in place.

Step 7: Use exercise as a silver bullet of good health

For someone who has never been an exercise aficionado, like with dieting, it evokes feelings of dread. But, truthfully, for most regular exercisers, it becomes something they love doing. This is because it has so many benefits that not doing it leaves you feeling the difference in your life.

The role of exercise in fighting diabetes

The most obvious reason to exercise is to control your weight. While it's true that dieting alone is sufficient to lose weight, exercise makes weight management much more sustainable in the long run, and weight loss much easier in the short term.

If you are what you eat, then it's also true that you are what you do. If you train your body, you will be stronger, healthier and happier guaranteed. That's why exercise is the silver bullet of good health.

Why exercise is one of the best things you can do for yourself

It releases happy hormones

Ever heard of runner's high? It's a real thing, and it doesn't only apply to runners. Any type of exercise produces a natural high that leaves you feeling great afterwards. This is because it prompts the release of endorphins. It quite literally makes you happier.

It's good for the brain

We were made to move. It's one of the main functions of the brain. Exercise has been shown to increase memory and thinking skills.

It's good for the heart

Cardiovascular exercise strengthens the heart and lungs.

It's good for the body

Spending most of your time sitting, as you would if you have a desk job, is very bad for the body, the muscles and the spine. We eventually develop weak postures and weak, atrophied muscles. Things like chronic back pain are attributable to this in many cases, either because you have weak stomach muscles that force that back muscles to take strain to help keep you upright, or because the glutes and hamstrings become shortened and tight, also causing the back to take strain.

It prevents injury

When your muscles are strong and limber, you are less likely to get seriously injured if you fall or perform strenuous activity. It also offers better protection for the joints.

It's good for longevity

When muscles are left unused, they become atrophied, and as we become older, we start to lose muscle mass and bone density. Eventually, this leads to conditions like osteoarthritis and osteoporosis, and the need for knee and hip replacements. Keeping the muscles strong helps with balance and co-ordination, reducing incidences of falling down in the elderly, which is why exercise isn't just a short-term fix to lose weight, it should be a life-long pursuit.

It ups the metabolism

Muscle is metabolically expensive, meaning that to retain it, grow it and move it, the body needs more calories. This results in a much higher basal metabolic rate. In other words, you are burning more calories even when you are sitting around doing nothing when you add some muscle mass.

It makes everyday life easier

Functional fitness means the activities you do during the day, like carrying groceries or climbing stairs, are much easier.

It ups the energy levels

Simply put: the more you do, the more you want to do.

How much is enough?

The recommended weekly time spent exercising is 150 minutes. This translates into about 30 minutes a day during the workweek.

More is not necessarily better with exercise, and overdoing it can stunt progress because your muscles need time to heal afterwards. In essence, you don't want to go over an hour, six days a week. This leaves us with a window of 30 to 50 minutes per session, five to six days a week.

The recovery phase of exercise is just as important as the actual exercise, so make sure to get those eight hours of sleep, drink lots of water and eat a nutrient-dense diet to optimise recovery.

Types of exercise

Cardio and HIIT

There is some hot debate about which is more efficient: high intensity interval training (HIIT) or steady state cardio (elliptical, jogging, cycling). HIIT can be very demanding on the muscles, so it's usually not a good idea to do it on consecutive days. When you're doing strength training as well, it can become harder for the body to recover. This is where steady state cardio is useful. However, some may find that lots of cardio can negatively effect muscle gain. Find a good balance that works for you, and always listen to your body. While it's good to push yourself, pushing too hard won't get you any results – you can sustain an injury or over-train, leading to negative effects on your health.

Strength training

As mentioned before, bigger muscles mean a faster metabolism. Strength is a must for any fitness routine. Traditionally, women avoid lifting weights, as they fear getting bulky, but this is a myth. Since women don't naturally produce much testosterone (which you must have to build muscle) and they also aren't really strong enough to lift that much anyway, they don't suddenly become muscled specimens of the Swarzenegger calibre, especially without supplementation.

Fast-paced strength training routines can become quite demanding on the cardiovascular system and in fact be like a cardio session. Plus they also burn a lot of calories, depending on how heavy you're lifting.

Strength training should be well rounded, as just focusing on some muscles and ignoring others can lead to imbalances. Your best bet is buying a programme to follow, or finding a free one online. If you're going to the gym, you could also hire a trainer.

Yoga and Pilates

To top off a well-rounded exercise routine with cardio/HIIT and strength training, add some Pilates or yoga.

Flexibility, co-ordination and range of motion are just as important as fitness and strength, and just as essential to keep the body supple enough to avoid injury in daily life and while exercising.

Putting it all together

Generally, a good routine will include two to three total body strength routines or two upper, two lower and one core routine per week. This can be topped off with some lighter cardio and HIIT. Remember to take at least one rest day a week, or more if you're feeling very sore.

It's important to note that this is just a general guideline – and you don't need to force yourself into a rigid exercise regimen. Take it week by week and see what you feel like. Exercise should not be a punishment, and even just 10 minutes a day will have benefits for you.

Step 8: Get some sweet, sweet sleep

Sleep is the body's me-time. This is where your brain gets a chance to switch off its focus on the outside world and focus instead on the body. There are many important processes that take place during this time, and good uninterrupted sleep of seven to nine hours every night is health therapy in itself.

Here are some benefits of good sleep:

Weight management

Getting little sleep has been linked to obesity in both adults and children – it's one of the biggest risk factors.

This is because sleep influences your hormones, most noticeably your cortisol levels (the stress hormone). When you get more sleep, your body has lower levels of cortisol. Elevated levels of cortisol are associated with various health issues, including weight gain and inability to lose weight.

Insulin sensitivity

Good sleep is also known to improve insulin sensitivity – the opposite of insulin resistance!

Immune supporter

Recent studies have found that people who get their eight hours are less likely to get sick – and less likely to get depressed.

Appetite suppressant

When you sleep badly or not much at all, you have a bigger appetite the next day and more cravings for bad foods (that means processed carbs). This is because insulin is not the only hormone affected by sleep. When you don't sleep, leptin (the hormone that makes you feel full) decreases and ghrelin (the hormone that makes you feel hungry) increases.

Recovery time

When you work out doing strength training or HIIT, your muscle fibres tear and your body has to repair them again. Most of this happens during sleep. After your body has healed its muscles, they come back bigger and stronger.

Step 9: Let off some steam

Stress plays a big role in our lives, and all the ways in which it affects the body aren't known, but we do know that it can drastically affect health – and lead to stubborn body fat that just won't go away.

While exercise and sleep alone are excellent for easing stress, there are also some other ways, like taking little breaks from work, listening to music or watching something funny online.

Most importantly though, make sure to take extended breaks like holidays or weekends away, and switch off completely during these. This will assist in keeping those cortisol levels under control.

Step 10: Stay clued up

As type-2 diabetes continues to recruit more members, it's becoming a priority among health professionals, and new research is being revealed all the time. It's in your best interest to keep up to date with all the recent developments, and there are so many channels through which to do just that.

Information is so readily available these days. You can google your heart out on anything you desire, and the latest seminars on diabetes are all being uploaded to YouTube. Knowledge is power, so get some!

Step 11: Look at other approaches

It's very obvious at this point that changing your diet is the base of reversing type-2 diabetes. Besides the low-carb approach, studies have indicated the vegans have a significantly lower risk of diabetes than meat eaters – as well as obesity and other diseases. This is thought to be because consuming meat, eggs and dairy means consuming the hormones in those animals as well – and these can throw out our own hormonal levels. Especially because animals bred for consumption are injected with growth hormones so they grow quicker.

The most common question about vegan and vegetarian diets is where does the protein come from? All plants have all three macros, just in smaller amounts. Eating a good variety will ensure that you get all of the essential amino acids in protein in sufficient amounts. Foods like legumes and quinoa are especially high in protein, and even some veggies like spinach, so make sure to eat lots of them. If you're worried about consuming enough protein, it's advisable to supplement with vegan protein powder. Many of them contain as much as 15g of protein per serving.

It's also necessary to supplement vitamin B12 if you don't consume animal products, but since your body naturally stores this, it's not an immediate deficiency that you need to worry about.

Here's a list of plant-based foods that are high in protein:

Vegan-friendly foods high in protein	
Beans Beans, beans, the magical fruit! These are a staple of any self-respecting vegan: they're kind of like the vegan version of meat. The list of bean types goes on and on. Many of them go around the 9g of protein per 100g mark. That's about 15g per cup.	**Quinoa** Quinoa is a complete protein, one of very few in the plant foods crowd. This means it contains all of the essential amino acids in good quantities. 9g of protein per cup.
Peas 5g of protein per 100g. Not bad!	**Chickpeas** Also known as garbanzo beans, these little things can have as much as 19g of protein per 100g! Lovely in salads.

Step 12: Pay attention to your body

Once you've adjusted to a low-carb diet and gotten rid of processed foods, you'll notice how much better you feel. And also how certain foods affect you. Start paying attention to this. You might find it helpful to keep a food diary that lists the foods you eat every day, as well as how you felt that day.

For instance, some types of veggies may be upsetting to your stomach. If you keep track of what you eat, you can pin down the culprit. Similarly, some find that dairy doesn't work that well for digestion and causes bloating.

At least for the first few months, weigh the foods you eat and log the exact amount of carbs you're getting in. Compare this with your blood-sugar levels and see how the amount of carbs you're eating affects you. There can be a dramatic difference between 20g and 60g of carbs, for instance.

Sample of a food diary:

Monday		
Total calories: **Carbs:** **Fat:** **Protein:**	Exercise: Sleep: Water consumed:	*How did you feel today?*

Chapter 3
Customise your plan - maintenance

All together, the 12 steps listed in the previous chapter map out the approach to start taking control of your diabetes. However, it's up to you to assimilate them into your life for the long run. Ultimately, this is a lifestyle, and diabetes could come back. It's a marathon, not a sprint. While the shorter term goal is to reverse diabetes, the longer term goal is to be healthy. And there may be times you slip up or experience what feels like steps backward, but in being consistent over time you will unlock the way to good health. Falling off the wagon is part and parcel of this journey, but it's your ability to get back on that will determine your ultimate success.

We're all different, and our bodies will respond differently to different foods and types of exercise. Find what works for you. Customise this plan to suit your life and goals. Pay attention to how you feel, and keep what makes you feel good, and take out what doesn't.

Conclusion

Now that you've got all this new information – doing something with it. The ball is in your court.

Good luck!

Thank you again for downloading this book!

If you would like another book in a similar category, please visit my author page at amazon.com/author/joshuanathan

Finally, if you enjoyed this book, please take the time to share your thoughts and post a review on Amazon, It'd be greatly appreciated!

Now go live your life to the fullest – and relish every moment of it!

Thank you and good luck!

http://www.mellowzoo.com

Scroll down for previews to other books we think will benefit you!

PREVIEW OF: "TIME MANAGEMENT: 12 SIMPLE TIME MANAGEMENT STEPS TO BETTER FOCUS, FASTER PROGRESS AND OPTIMAL RESULTS"

"Productivity is not just about doing more, it is about creating more impact with less work."

– Prima Malik

Time is a finite commodity; we have only the allotted number of hours in a day
to get things done. And if you're anything like the millions of people out there
trying to keep up in this always-on, always-connected digital age, it might
seem like those hours just aren't enough.

But what if you changed the way you used those hours? The simple fact is
that successful people manage their time better. It's not about trying to do
more, it's about streamlining what you're already doing – focusing enough
time on the right tasks – and in that way opening up more time for other

pursuits, like those things you've always wanted to do, but can never get
around to.

That's the topic this book explores: harnessing good time management,
sharper focus and correct planning to make every 24 hours as productive as
they can possibly be. It's really that easy. You just need to change your
approach.

So if you're ready to super-charge what you're really capable of accomplishing every day, let's get started!

Download on my author page on amazon
amazon.com/author/joshuanathan

PREVIEW OF: "MINDFULNESS: BE PRESENT, SAVOUR EVERY MOMENT AND LIVE A HAPPIER LIFE IN 12 SIMPLE STEPS"

"Most humans are never fully present in the now, because unconsciously they believe that the next moment must be more important than this one. But then you miss your whole life, which is never not now. And that's a revelation for some people: to realise that your life is only ever now."

– Eckhart Tolle

Think about how much time you spend walking around on auto-pilot, only ever paying attention when someone says your name. What's happening around you right now – the sounds, the smells, the atmosphere. Have you noticed any of it?

It's time to become **mindful** – noticing, experiencing and appreciating the present more; learning to savour the moment and create more memorable ones; reinforcing bonds with the people in your life by paying attention to them; taking care of your body and mind the way they deserve; and easing the stress of everyday living by increasing your understanding of yourself.

This book is an aid to help you snap out of it for good, and actually live in the moment. After all, the only time that really exists is the present. It's all you have, and all you ever will have. You cannot change the past; and the future is forever out of reach. Life is such a precious gift – stop letting it pass you by.

Try these 12 simple steps, and I guarantee you'll walk out of the experience with a new perspective – and hopefully as a happier, less stressed and more present human being, who'll live a fuller life as a consequence.

So are you ready to live in the moment? Let's get started!

Download on my author page on amazon
amazon.com/author/joshuanathan

PREVIEW OF: "SLEEP SECRETS: 12 SIMPLE TIME MANAGEMENT STEPS TO BETTER FOCUS, FASTER PROGRESS AND OPTIMAL RESULTS"

And so it begins

It's 2 o'clock on a Monday morning. You're still awake. Wide awake. Staring at the ceiling yet again, worrying every 10 minutes about how much time you have left to sleep before you have to get up for work. The more you try to close your eyes and concentrate on falling asleep, the harder it seems to be. It's a vicious circle. You're exhausted and frustrated, but your brain just won't 'click' off.

I've been there, for 6 months I relied on the little sleep I got to keep functioning. If I managed 4 hours it was a great night, but when it started dropping to 2 hours, then 1 hour, then 20 minutes, I knew I had to do something! Anything! I was in a state of turmoil, and it seemed as though nothing was helping which simply made my frustration worse. It started affecting my mood, my work and my relationships. I had to find a way. I took months trying to figure out what it was that was keeping me awake, I was willing to try anything out of sheer desperation.

Then one day I got it right.

If like me, you are at that point where you are feeling frustrated and you just need to sleep, then this book is for you. I have taken the time to meticulously compile everything I've tried into one small, easy to follow guide in the hopes that my experiences could somehow help you. You will learn how to give yourself every advantage to fall asleep, from getting your environment ready to monitoring your patterns with a sleep log and trying various techniques on how to relax a busy mind.

The purpose of this book is purely to help you figure out what is keeping you
awake and how we can possibly fix that together.

So if you're ready for some serious shuteye then let's get started!

Download on my author page on amazon
amazon.com/author/joshuanathan